Food Works

Frederick Mickel Huck

authorHOUSE®

AuthorHouse™
1663 Liberty Drive, Suite 200
Bloomington, IN 47403
www.authorhouse.com
Phone: 1-800-839-8640

First published by AuthorHouse   3/6/2009

ISBN: 978-1-4343-4659-9 (sc)

Library of Congress Control Number: 2009900760

Printed in the United States of America
Bloomington, Indiana

This book is printed on acid-free paper.

This Book is Dedicated to

ROBERT E. MENZIE

INEZ A. MENZIE

DONALD WALTER HUCK

AURA VICTORIA HUCK

INSPIRED BY

DOCTOR EDE KOENIG

And Special Thanks to

SANDRA MOONEY

MATT MOONEY

Table of Contents

Introduction

The American Diet

What most people call food today amounts to the perfect definition of junk food, which is heavily altered and changed so much, that very little nutritional value remains. With white sugar, oils, and animal products consumed in abundance, it's no wonder that the end results bring about the body malfunctioning at epidemic levels. It's considered normal to be sick nowadays with added medications, convenience foods, and fad diet plans. When the body lacks the nutrition it needs, it cannot work the way it should or function, which ends up affecting one's physical and mental state. A person who is not healthy is settling for less or for a lower quality of life. It's also very expensive to be sick, with numerous doctor visits, lab tests, and surgical procedures. I find it much easier to do what is right for the body, which starts with real and healthy delicious foods. This book contains many examples and ideas that will help replace the foods that are considered junk.

Fourteen Days of Meals

The purpose of this fourteen-day meal plan is to illustrate that starvation does not happen when following the plan. Instead of listing the fruit on a daily log every day, I just list here approximately what fruit was eaten. For the last two years, I have reversed my two meals, where the larger meal of the day was consumed first, and the second mostly a raw meal later in the day. Prior to eating breakfast, generally a half hour after I wake, I drink a quart of warm water with two teaspoons of lemon juice, one tablespoon of inland sea water, and one tablespoon of silver mineral water.

Approximately five pounds of fruit is consumed daily, and the fruit varies according to the seasons of the year.

For dinner, I usually have a salad, which consists of:

red head lettuce

three radishes cut small

one long green onion, cut small

one-third of a carrot, cut small

half of an avocado

half of a celery stalk, cut small

six tbsp. of lemon juice

approximately one tablespoon of Bragg Liquid Aminos

up to twelve ounces or more of two different kinds of hot sauce as tolerated

bread, crackers, or corn tortillas

These fourteen days referred to a fruit meal which is available raw fruit in season. My fruit meal consisted of three different colors of apples, twelve cherries, one nectarine, one mango, and one slice of pineapple, one slice of cantaloupe, eight green grapes, one apricot, and one peach. In addition, I also eat eight raw Brazil nuts, six apricot nuts, one teaspoon of sunflower seeds, one teaspoon of pumpkin seeds, two capsules of calcium, and two capsules of magnesium.

Fourteen Days of Meals

Day 1

Breakfast—Lunch:	Salad, 10 corn tortillas, 2 stuffed bell peppers, 6 ounces of herbs and garlic rice
Dessert:	6 ounces of orange ice cream
Dinner:	Raw nuts (mixed), one large waffle, approximately 5 pounds of fresh fruit

Fourteen Days of Meals

Day 2

Breakfast—Lunch:	Salad, approximately one-third pound of wheat crackers, approximately 2 pounds of Spanish pasta
Dessert:	One-quarter pound of apricot bars
Dinner:	Raw nuts (mixed), approximately 5 pounds of fresh fruit, 6 ounces of Habanera rice-

Fourteen Days of Meals

Day 3

Breakfast—Lunch:	Salad, approximately one-third pound of Lavash Tonir bread, 3 egg rolls, 6 ounces of Chinese rice
Dessert:	One-quarter pound of Gene Koenig English toffee candy bar
Dinner:	Raw nuts (mixed), approximately 5 pounds of fresh fruit, large bowl of popcorn

Fourteen Days of Meals

Day 4

Breakfast—Lunch: Salad, approximately one-third pound of Lavash Tonir bread, 24 ounces of vegetable soup, 6 ounces of Cajun rice

Dessert: One-quarter pound of carob salt water taffy

Dinner: Raw nuts (mixed), approximately 5 pounds of fresh fruit, 2 slices of Ezekiel bread with cherry jam.

Fourteen Days of Meals

Day 5

Breakfast—Lunch:	Salad, 2 slices of soymilk cornbread, 12 ounces of black-eyed peas, 12 ounces of baked brown rice
Dessert:	One-quarter pound of Donald W. Huck coconut cookies
Dinner:	Raw nuts (mixed), approximately 5 pounds of fresh fruit, 6 ounces of Cajun dry-roasted nuts

Fourteen Days of Meals

Day 6

Breakfast—Lunch:	Salad, approximately one-third pound of wheat crackers, 4 pocket pizzas
Dessert:	One-quarter pound of Robert E. Menzie walnut pie
Dinner:	Raw nuts (mixed), approximately 5 pounds of fresh fruit, 6 ounces of Puerto Rican rice

Fourteen Days of Meals

Day 7

Breakfast—Lunch:	Salad, 10 corn tortillas, 3 pocket bean burritos, 6 ounces of Spanish rice
Dessert:	6 ounces of raisin ice cream
Dinner:	Raw nuts (mixed), approximately 5 pounds of fresh fruit, 6 ounces of salted roasted nut mix

Fourteen Days of Meals

Day 8

Breakfast—Lunch: Salad, approximately one-third pound of Lavash Tonir bread, pot pie, 6 ounces of Texas rice

Dessert: One-quarter pound of pecan fudge

Dinner: Raw nuts (mixed), approximately 5 pounds of fresh fruit, 6 ounces of black bean rice

Fourteen Days of Meals

Day 9

Breakfast—Lunch: 2 taco salads, 6 ounces of herb and garlic baked rice

Dessert: One-quarter pound of cherry tofu cookies

Dinner: Raw nuts (mixed), approximately 5 pounds of fresh fruit, large bowl of oatmeal

Fourteen Days of Meals

Day 10

Breakfast—Lunch: Salad, one-third pound of Lavash Tonir bread, approximately one and a half pounds of enchiladas, 6 ounces of Habanera rice.

Dessert: 6 ounces of carob ice cream

Dinner: Raw nuts (mixed), approximately 5 pounds of fresh fruit, one large waffle.

Fourteen Days of Meals

Day 11

Breakfast—Lunch:	Salad, one-third pound of Lavash Tonir bread, 2 slices of garlic bread, 12 ounces of Chinese rice
Dessert:	One-quarter pound of peach pie
Dinner:	Raw nuts (mixed), approximately 5 pounds of fresh fruit, 6 ounces of Habanera dry-roasted nut mix

Fourteen Days of Meals

Day 12

Breakfast—Lunch:	Salad, one-third pound of wheat crackers, 2 slices of soymilk cornbread, 12 ounces of lentils, 12 ounces of baked brown rice
Dessert:	One-quarter pound of coconut roma caramel candy
Dinner:	Raw nuts (mixed), approximately 5 pounds of fresh fruit, 6 ounces of onion dry roasted nuts

Fourteen Days of Meals

Day 13

Breakfast—Lunch:	Salad, one-third pound of Lavash Tonir wheat bread, twenty-four ounces of potato and cabbage stew, six ounces of green jalapeno rice mix
Dessert:	One-fourth pound of Aura Victoria Huck Salt water taffy
Dinner:	Raw nuts (mixed), approximately 5 pounds of fresh fruit 6 ounces of onion dry roasted nuts

Fourteen Days of Meals

Day 14

Breakfast—Lunch:	Salad, one-third pound of wheat crackers, 2 tamales, 12 ounces of Texas rice
Dessert:	One-quarter pound of walnut fudge
Dinner:	Raw nuts (mixed), approximately 5 pounds of fresh fruit, 6 ounces of black-eyed pea rice

Setting up the Pantry Plus

Popcorn - it should be dry popcorn

Bragg Liquid Aminos – a natural soy sauce. It must be refrigerated after opening. Can be used for salads, beans, and rice or pasta recipes Coconut powder – a fine powder used for cooking

Tofu – (I recommend Mori-Nu Tofu). Ingredients: water, soybeans, gluconlastone, and calcium chloride

Sage, celery seeds, dill weed, ground marjoram, turmeric, whole caraway seeds

Soymilk – Ingredients: organic whole soybeans, rice syrup, filtered water

Vitamix – or a blender

Pure vanilla – no alcohol

Puffed rice and puffed corn

Maple syrup – 100 percent

Roma coffee – Ingredients: roasted malt, barley, roasted barley, roasted chicory

Carob – a natural chocolate substitute

Tapioca – for thickening; grind into a fine powder

Corn tortillas – brand name Mi Rancho. Ingredients: water, corn, and lime

Canned green olives – Ingredients: olives, water, and salt

Tomato paste – tomato only, can be bought in a can (no salt)

Cereals – stay away from any sugar, any oil, and any fructose; look for whole grains only

Oatmeal – old-fashioned Quaker oats, 100 percent whole grain and natural only

Ezekiel bread – 4:9 brand; they make a sesame seed wheat, cinnamon, rye bread

Organic Sucanat Sugar – natural certified sweetener (brown color only). The brand is Natural Touch: Wholesome Sweetener

Teflon cooking trays – stainless steel pots, pans, or glass

Cookie mats – parchment paper

100 percent durum wheat semolina – Ingredients: niacin, ferrous lactate, (iron), thiamin, mononitrate, riboflavin, and folic acid

Oregano, ground thyme

Corn – fresh or frozen (no salt)

Peas – fresh or frozen (no salt)

Pineapple – fresh or in a can – Ingredients: 100 percent pineapple, pineapple juice, water, and certified pineapple juice concentrate

Bio-salt – inland sea water

Lemons – fresh

Oatmeal

Whole cornmeal

Corn flour

Apricot pits – the nut inside the pit, raw

Brazil nuts – raw

Pumpkin seeds – raw

Paprika

Garlic powder

Almonds – raw

Sunflower seeds – raw

Parsley flakes

Red chilies – fresh or dry flakes

Whole caraway seeds

Celery seeds

Ground ginger

Chili powder

Cayenne pepper

Italian seasonings

Cinnamon – ground

Cumin

Onion – dried

Dry yeast – only used to make dough rise

Whole summer savory leaf

Pristine oil – used instead of toothpaste, because toothpaste is composed of sand, fluoride and other chemicals

Magnesium: (must have kelp) dulse rue, black walnut – whole, black walnut leaf, butcher's broom, oat straw, calcium, horsetail, comfrey, dandelion root, alfalfa, oat straw, parsley root, and lobelia; these ingredients are all natural and based on herbs

Water Pic for dental hygiene

Corning ware dishes

Hydrogen peroxide 3 percent

Shampoo, deodorant, shaving cream. Aubrey products can be found in any health-food store

Ozone generator – for drinking water and cleaning fruits and vegetables and for spraying pots and pans, dishes, cooking equipment, and cleaning hands

Toilet tissues and paper towels, use white only; colors have toxins

Recipe 37

Any Fruit Cookies (Peach, Cherry, Apricot)

Directions:

Mix the following in a bowl:

1 cup almond butter

½ cup maple syrup

½ cup tofu

1/4 tsp. Bio-salt

½ tsp. vanilla

1½ cups chopped walnuts

2½ cups sifted whole wheat pastry flour

Mix the dough; roll by hand into small round balls.   Press your thumb to form an indentation on the centers, and then add the fruit. (Can be jam if 100 percent fruit) in the indentations.

Place cookies on trays using parchment paper or cookie mat.

Place in 375-degree oven for 15 minutes.

Recipe 38

Special Pie Crust

Directions:

Mix in a Vitamix or blender the following:

1 cup almonds

1/3 tsp. Bio-salt

1 cup oatmeal

1/4 cup coconut

In the actual pie dish, add 4 tbsp. maple syrup, and mix all of the above.

Form into a crust.

When using fruit for the filling, fill the shell.

Bake for 45 minutes.

Recipe 39 ———————————————————

Pumpkin Pie

Directions:

Place into a Vitamix or blender the following:

1/4 tsp. allspice

3/4 tsp. cinnamon

1 tsp. Bio-salt

1 cup maple syrup

½ cup Sucanat sugar

1 tsp. vanilla

½ cup cashews

1 29 ounce can pumpkin (enough for two pies)

See special pie crust recipe number 38, for pie shell.

Bake at 350 degrees for 20 minutes.

Recipe 40

Parvin Malek Carob Pie

Directions:

Place in a Vitamix or blender the following:

1 brick tofu

1 cup maple syrup

1 cup almond butter

¼ cup carob powder

¼ cup Roma coffee powder

½ cup Sucanat sugar

½ cup whole-wheat pastry flour

See special pie crust recipe number 38.

Place all of the above in an uncooked pie shell.

Bake at 350 degrees for 20 minutes.

Recipe 41

Almond Butter Cookies #2

Mix in a bowl the following:

3/4 cup plus 4 tbsp. almond butter

½ cup maple syrup

1/4 cup tofu

½ cup Sucanat sugar

Place the above in a bowl and mix by hand. When mixed, add the following:
1-1/3 cups sifted whole-wheat pastry flour.
Can be mixed 24 hours in advance and placed in refrigerator; dough will be very soft.

Take out of refrigerator and form the cookie with a spoon on cookie tray lined with parchment paper or a cookie mat.

Bake at 375 degrees for 15 minutes.

Recipe 42 ———————————————————————

Carob Filling

Place into a bowl and mix the following:

4 tbsp. almond butter

1/4 cup carob

2 cups Sucanat sugar

1/4 cup soymilk or water

Mix and add to doughnuts when cool.

(For the inside of doughnuts or for cake frostings.)

Recipe 43 —————————

Evelyn Ann Menzie Old-fashioned Glaze (For Top Of Doughnuts Or Cakes)

Directions:

Mix in a small bowl:

2 tbsp. maple syrup

3 tbsp. soy milk

2 cups Sucanat sugar

Doughnuts or cake must be cool before adding the glaze.

Recipe 44

Pineapple Pie

Mix in a pan and boil for one hour and ½ on warm:

1/4 tsp. Bio-salt

2 cans pineapple (crushed)

1 cup Sucanat sugar

1 cup maple syrup

    Then
    Add 3 tbsp. tapioca flour*

Stir and continue to boil for 30 minutes, stirring occasionally. For pie shell, see special pie crust recipe #38.

Pour this mixture into pie shell.

Return to oven for 45 minutes. Bake at 350 degrees.

* Place tapioca in a blender until ground into flour.

For firmer filling, boil for 30 more minutes.

Recipe 45 ——————————————

Butter Cookies

Mix in a Vitamix or blender the following:

2 tsp. rose water

1 tsp. vanilla

3 cups maple syrup

1 tsp. Bio-salt

3 cups almond butter (add one cup at a time)

Pour all these ingredients in a bowl.

Add 4 cups whole-wheat pastry flour.

Stir and let sit until thick.

Place on tray lined with parchment paper or a cookie mat.

Bake at 375 degrees for 10 minutes.

Recipe 46 ——————————————————————————

Sucanat Cookies
(See Butter Cookie Recipe #45)

When re-rolling the cookie dough, add sugar and flour to floured board.

You will need 1 to 2 pounds of Sucanat sugar.

You can use round cookie cutter or any basic shape cutter.

Bake 13 minutes if cookie is thick.

Bake 10 minutes if cookie is thin.

Bake at 375 degrees.

Mix dough the night before, place in a covered bowl, and refrigerate.

Recipe 47 ──────────────────

Inez A. Menzie Carob Coconut Cookies

Mix in a large bowl the following:

6 cups maple syrup

2 tsp. almond butter

1 tsp. Bio-salt

3 tbsp. Roma powder

3 tbsp. carob

2 cups oatmeal flour *

4 cups shredded coconut

5 cups sifted whole-wheat pastry flour

Stir and form into cookies.

Place on cookie tray lined with parchment paper or a cookie mat.

This cookie is very large and makes 3 dozen cookies. Use 3 trays, 12 per tray.

Bake in oven at 325 degrees for 25 minutes.

* Oatmeal flour is made by putting 100 percent whole oats in a blender.

Recipe 48 _____

Turnovers

(Any fruit: pineapple, apricot, cherry, peach)

For dough, use the butter cookie recipe; see number 45.

Make dough the night before and place covered in refrigerator.

The next day, make thin squares, 5 inches by 5 inches.

Place the fruit in the center and fold over.

Make holes with fork on top of each one.

Place on cookie sheet lined with parchment paper or cookie mat.

See any pie recipe for the inside fillings of the turnovers.

Bake at 425 degrees for 15 to 20 minutes.

Recipe 49

Golden Macaroons

Add to large bowl and mix:

2 cups grated carrots

6 cups maple syrup

2 tsp. almond butter

4 cups coconut

1 tsp. Bio-salt

Mix well, and then add 5 cups of sifted whole-wheat pastry flour.

Let stand for 3 to 4 hours, if cookie dough is too thin.

Then form into cookies and place on tray lined with parchment paper or cookie mat.

Bake at 325 degrees for 30 minutes.

Recipe 50

Oriental Crunch

Place in a bowl and mix by hand the following:

1 tsp. vanilla

1 cup almond butter

½ tsp. Bio-salt

2 tbsp. Roma powder

1 cup maple syrup

1 cup Sucanat sugar

¼ cup carob powder

Continue to stir and add:

3 cups whole-wheat pastry flour

Place in a pie dish lined with parchment paper. Sprinkle ½ cup chopped almonds on the top. Press into the dough.

Bake for 20 minutes at 375 degrees.

Recipe 51 ——————————————

Pineapple Candy

In a large bowl, mix the following by hand:

8 tbsp. wheat germ

2 cups chopped walnuts

2 tsp. Bio-salt

2 tsp. vanilla

4 tsp. flaxseed meal

6 cups maple syrup

Continue to stir, and then add:

12 cups dried pineapple, cut small

Mix and add 4 cups whole-wheat pastry flour.

Add 4 cups oatmeal flour.

Place ingredients on parchment paper-lined 13 x 9-inch glass dish.

Bake at 200 degrees for two and a half hours.

Recipe 52 ————————————————————————

Carob Doughnuts

Place in a Vitamix or blender the following and mix:

1-1/3 cups soymilk

One cup Sucanat Sugar

One cup maple syrup

One tbsp. Almond Butter

½ tsp. Bio-salt

½ cup Tofu

One third cup Carob powder

Mix

Pour ingredients into a bowl and add two cups sifted whole-wheat pastry flour.

Mix one tbsp. yeast in ¼ cup warm water; let dough sit and rise.
Pour into doughnut molds or lined cupcake pans.

Bake at 400 degrees for 10 minutes.

If adding frosting or glaze, make sure doughnuts are cool.

Recipe 53 ———————————

Lemon Doughnuts

Place in a Vitamix or blender the following:

1 cup maple syrup

1 tbsp. almond butter

2 tsp. Bio-salt

½ cup tofu

1 tbsp. lemon juice

1 cup soymilk

Mix and pour into a bowl.

Mix 1 tbsp. yeast in ¼ cup warm water.   Add 2 cups whole-wheat pastry flour.

Mix and stir.

Pour into doughnut molds or lined cupcake pan.

Bake at 400 degrees for 10 minutes.

If adding frosting or glazes make sure the doughnuts are cool.

Recipe 54 ───────────────────

Grain Pizza

In a large bowl, mix the following:

2 tsp. Sucanat sugar

1 tsp. almond butter

½ tsp. Bio-salt

2 tbsp. cornmeal

2 tbsp. sifted barley flour

¼ cup oatmeal flour

¼ cup sifted rye flour

1½ cups sifted whole-wheat pastry flour

Mix 1 tbsp. yeast in 1 cup lukewarm water and add to a large bowl.

Mix and knead by hand for approximately 5 to 10 minutes; dough should be elastic. If not, add water, a teaspoon at a time until moist.

Place in a covered bowl, and place in a warm area for 20 minutes, then roll into a ball.

Place into a parchment paper-lined pan.

Form into a circle. Press into a 9 x 9-inch round pan.

Bake for 15 to 20 minutes at 425 degrees.

See pizza sauce recipe for toppings.

Recipe 55

Cornmeal Pizza

In a large bowl, mix the following:

1½ cups sifted whole-wheat pastry flour

¼ cup cornmeal

¼ tsp. Bio-salt

1 tsp. almond butter

½ to 2/3 cup lukewarm water, mixed with 1 tbsp. yeast

Mix all ingredients and knead by hand for approximately 5 to 10 minutes. The dough must be elastic; if not, add 1 tsp. water until the dough is moist.

Place in a covered bowl, put bowl in warm area for 15 to 20 minutes; dough should double in size. Knead for another 3 minutes, and roll into a ball. Place ball on parchment paper-lined 9 x 9-inch pan. Press dough into pan to form pizza.

Bake at 425 degrees for 15 to 20 minutes.

See pizza sauce recipe for toppings.

Recipe 56

Carob Brownies

Mix in a large bowl the following:

6 cups maple syrup

2 tsp. almond butter

1 tbsp. Bio-salt

4 tbsp. carob powder

4 tbsp. Roma powder

2 tbsp. soymilk

1 tsp. vanilla

6 cups ground walnuts

4 cups sifted whole-wheat pastry flour

Mix and place all ingredients in a 9 x 13-inch glass dish lined with parchment paper.

Bake at 350 degrees for 50 minutes.

Use the toothpick test to make sure the center is cooked.

Let cool and cut into squares.

Recipe 57 ————————————————————————

Robert E. Menzie Walnut Pie
For crust see special pie crust recipe No. 38.

In a small bowl, mix by hand the following:

1 tsp. vanilla

1 cup Sucanat sugar

½ cup almond butter

½ cup tofu

Mix and then add:

2 cups chopped walnuts

Stir again, add to uncooked pie crust, level with a spoon into the pie shell, and then pour one cup maple syrup on top.

Bake at 375 degrees for 25 minutes.

Recipe 58

Apricot Coconut Walnut Squares

The crust:

In a large bowl, mix the following:

2 cups maple syrup

2 cups almond butter

Stir; add 2 cups sifted whole-wheat pastry flour.

The dough will be sticky; use spoon and knife to spread the dough on a cookie sheet lined with parchment paper.   Do not use a flat cookie sheet; use a traditional cookie sheet with four sides.

Bake at 350 degrees for 20 to 25 minutes.

Topping:

Place in a Vitamix or blender the following:

1 brick tofu

1 tsp. vanilla

1 tsp. rose water

½ tsp. Bio-salt

2 Tsp. lemon juice

2 cups maple syrup

1 tsp. tapioca

Pour into a bowl; add 2 cups apricots, cut small.
Stir and add ½ cup whole-wheat pastry flour. Pour into a baked crust.

Add to topping:

1 cup coconut

4 cups ground walnuts

Bake at 350 degrees for 18 to 20 minutes.

Recipe 59

Pistachio Scones

In a Vitamix or blender, mix the following:

½ tsp. Bio-salt

½ cup almond butter

1 cup maple syrup

¼ cup tofu

1 tsp. lemon juice

1½ cups soymilk

Pour in a large bowl and add:

1 cup roasted pistachios

2 cups cornmeal

3 cups whole-wheat pastry flour

Mix and roll into 2 equal balls, then roll these balls into Sucanat sugar. Flatten the dough into a round circle; flatten it to approximately half an inch thick. Then cut into sections like a pie. Place the wedges on a cookie tray lined with parchment paper.

Makes 16 wedges

Bake 30 minutes at 350 degrees.

Recipe 60 _____

Egg Rolls

The following must be shredded and placed in a large pan:

12 radishes

4 cups carrots

2 bell peppers

Add:

6 tbsp. Bragg Liquid Aminos

1 tbsp. Bio-salt

Cut small and add to the same pan the following:

2 cups onions

4 cups of celery

8 cloves of garlic

4 cups of cabbage

> boil for five minutes and add 1 pound or 16 ounces of bean sprouts
> continue to mix and boil for three minutes, let cool completely
> wrap like bean burritos, place on trays
> bake 450 degrees for ten minutes
> yields, 36 egg rolls and requires four bags of bread (Lavash Tonir)

Recipe 61

Roasted- Salted Nuts

In a large bowl pour 4 cups of the following:

walnuts, almonds, pecans,

Stir and spray with Bragg Liquid Aminos, until thoroughly coated.

Add 1 tbsp. Bio-salt.

Stir and spray again with Bragg Liquid Aminos, then add 5 cups puffed corn.

Continue to spray with Bragg Liquid Aminos until all the mixture is coated.

Place in a cookie tray lined with parchment paper. Then turn the oven to 200 degrees for 12 hours or until dry.

Recipe 62 _____

Fudge Cup Cookie
For dough see butter cookie recipe #45

Roll out the dough; use a round cookie cutter circle 4 x 4 inches

cut a circle in the dough and place the circle lightly inside a paper cupcake holder, carefully place into a cupcake pan.

Place in oven for 10 minutes at 375 degrees.

For filling: See fudge sauce recipe #63

Then add to baked cookie. You can freeze any extra.

Recipe 63

Fudge Sauce

Place in a pan:

4 cups Sucanat sugar

¼ tsp. cinnamon

¼ cup carob powder

¼ cup almond butter

1½ cups chopped pecans

1 cup whole pecans

3 cups soymilk

1 tsp. vanilla

3 tbsp. maple syrup

Boil on warm for 45 to 60 minutes.

Use with butter cookie recipe #45
or fudge cupcake recipe #62

Recipe 64 ──────────────

Pineapple Cookies

Place in a Vitamix or a blender the following:

1 cup soymilk

1 tsp. vanilla

1 cup maple syrup

1 tsp. cinnamon

½ cup Sucanat sugar

1 tsp. Bio-salt

1 cup almond butter

½ cup tofu

Mix and pour into a large bowl and add 8 cups ground walnuts.

Add 12 cups dried pineapple, cut small.

Stir and add:

2½ cups sifted whole-wheat pastry flour.   Continue to mix by hand.

Form and place on a cookie sheet lined with parchment paper or a cookie mat.

Bake at 350 degrees for 20 minutes.

Recipe 65 ——————————————

Tamale Bean Pie

Cook in a pan the following ingredients for 15 to 20 minutes:

½ chopped onion

one six ounce can green olives (each cut in half)

3 cups tomatoes (cut small)

1 tbsp. chili powder

1   tsp. garlic powder

1 cup bell peppers (cut small)

1 tsp. Bio-salt

1 tbsp. Bragg Liquid Aminos

1 tbsp. lemon juice

1 tbsp. paprika powder

Continue to stir.

Add 32 ounces cooked red or pinto beans.

Continue to stir.

CRUST:

Place in a Vitamix or blender the following:

1½ cups soymilk

1 cup almond butter

Pour into a large bowl.

Add:

1 tsp. Bio-salt

6 cups frozen corn

2 cups cornmeal

Stir, and then place in a 9 x 13-inch glass dish, lined with parchment paper.

These are the ingredients for the crust, and it needs to be patted down to form a crust.

Dough will be sticky, so use the back of a spoon to form the edges of the pie crust.   Once the shell is formed, pour the ingredients from the pan into the shell.

Bake at 350 degrees for 35 minutes.

Recipe 66 _____

Nut Pie

THE CRUST:

In a bowl, mix the following:

1 tsp. rose water

2 tbsp. maple syrup

¼ tsp. Bio-salt

1½ cups almond butter

1½ to 2 cups whole-wheat pastry flour

Place in a glass dish.

Bake at 350 degrees for 10 minutes.

THE FILLING:

Place in a pan the following:

1 cup maple syrup

½ cup almond butter

1 cup dried fruit, cut small

Boil for 5 minutes on low, and then add the following to the pan:

1 cup roasted chopped almonds

1 cup roasted ground pecans

1 tbsp. carob

1 tbsp. Roma

Pour the ingredients from the pan into the crust.

Place in refrigerator for 2 hours before serving.

Recipe 67

Date-walnut Cookies/sandwich

In a Vitamix or blender, mix the following:

½ cup Sucanat sugar

¼ tsp. Bio-salt

1 tsp. vanilla

2 cups maple syrup

4 cups dates

Pour in a bowl.

For dough recipe, see butter cookie recipe #45.

Grind 2 to 3 cups walnuts.

Roll dough thin with a rolling pin.   With a round 2 inch cookie cutter, cut dough into circles. Place half a spoon of date mixture on the center of the circles. Sprinkle walnuts on top and then place another circle on top to form a sandwich. Press the edges together to seal the mixture together. Poke top with a toothpick or fork.

Bake at 375 degrees for 10 minutes.

Recipe 68

Caramelized Ginger Hazelnut Tart

CRUST:

In a bowl, mix the following:

4 tbsp. maple syrup

1 cup almond butter

¼ tsp. Bio-salt

1 tsp. vanilla

2 cups whole-wheat pastry flour

Mix. Place on a cookie sheet 12 x 17 inches, lined with parchment paper. The dough will be sticky; spread with a knife.

Bake at 350 degrees for 10 minutes.

FILLING:

In a pan, boil the following:

3 cups maple syrup

½ cup carob powder

½ cup dried fruit, cut small

4 tsp. ginger powder

4 cups hazelnuts, chopped (OR 2 cups walnuts and 2 cups hazelnuts)

Continue to boil for 10 minutes.

Add to the baked crust.

Place in oven at 400 degrees for 8 minutes.

Recipe 69

Papaya Cookies

Place in a Vitamix or blender the following:

1 cup soymilk

1 tsp. vanilla

1 cup maple syrup

1 tsp. cinnamon

½ cup Sucanat sugar

1 tsp. Bio-salt

1 cup almond butter

½ cup tofu

Pour into a large bowl.

Add 8 cups ground walnuts.
Add 12 cups dried papaya, cut small.

Stir and add:

2½ cups whole-wheat pastry flour

Continue to mix by hand.   Form and place cookies on cookie sheet lined with parchment paper or a cookie mat.

Bake at 350 degrees for 20 minutes.

Recipe 70 _____

Cajun Mixed Nuts

In a large bowl mix 4 cups of the following:

almonds

walnuts

pecans

   Spray with Bragg Liquid Aminos, until all the nuts are coated then add 1 tbsp. of the following:

onion powder

chili powder

garlic powder

paprika

Bio-salt

Spray again with Bragg Liquid Aminos and continue to stir.

   Add 3 to 5 cups puffed corn.

   Continue to stir and add more Bragg Liquid Aminos until all mixture is coated.

   Place on a cookie tray lined with parchment paper.

   Place in oven at 200 degrees for 12 hours or overnight.

Recipe 71

Taco Salad Shells

Use cut bread, burrito size or large enough to put into a shell mold.

Bake at 375 degrees for 8 to 10 minutes.

Note: Use Lavash Tonir Bread and taco shell mold, after baked.

Let cool and add:

beans
Bragg Liquid Aminos
lettuce
avocado
hot sauce
radish
lemon juice

Recipe 72 ──────────────

For Cake
Wedding-style Cake

One, two, three, cakes placed on top each other; use any the doughnut recipes; add 5 times the amount.   Make all the cakes from the same recipe.

Bake in oven 325 degrees:

6-inch for about 35 minutes.

12-inch for about 45 minutes.

16-inch for about 50 minutes.

Use toothpick test to see if center is done.

Recipe 73

Spanish Millet Casserole

In a large baking bowl place:

3 cups millet

12 cups water

Soak overnight. The next day, add the following to a pan and sauté for five minutes:

2 tsp. garlic powder

3 tsp. salsa

1 tsp. cumin

2 cups tomatoes cut small

1 large bell pepper, cut small

2 tbsp. Bragg Liquid Aminos

Place contents into the above large baking bowl and mix.

Bake at 350 degrees for 3 hours.

Recipe 74 ———————————————————————

Enchiladas

FILLING:

See Spanish millet recipe #73. Use the entire recipe; make this the day before. Once cool, place covered in refrigerator.

In a large pan, place the following:

25 - 30 tomatoes (cut small)

4 tsp. garlic powder

½ onion, chopped

4 tbsp. chili powder

2 tsp. Bio-salt

2 cups corn

1 six ounce can olives (cut each in half)

4 bell peppers (cut small)

Boil for 2 hours on low to warm, until sauce is thick, and then add Spanish millet recipe   and mix.

Topping Sauce

In a Vitamix place:

30 - 40 tomatoes

4 tsp. cumin

4 tsp. oregano

2 tsp. thyme

8 tsp. garlic powder

½ onion

2 tsp, Bio-salt

Boil for 2 hours on low, and set aside.

(This recipe requires 33 corn tortillas for enchilada wrap.)

Place 2 to 3 spoons of filling into corn tortilla and fold. Wrap and place in a glass baking dish (9 x 13 inches). Repeat process, add sauce to each layer, then when through, pour the outside sauce over the top, and sprinkle cut long green onions on top of enchiladas.

Bake at 350 degrees for 25 to 30 minutes.

Recipe 75

Carob Pie

Place in a Vitamix the following:

¼ cup plus 1 tbsp. tapioca

½ cup very warm water

Then add the following:

2 cups maple syrup

¼ tsp. Bio-salt

1 brick or 1 pound tofu

½ cup Roma

½ cup carob

For crust, see special pie crust recipe #38.

After pie crust is formed, bake 10 minutes at 350 degrees.

Then add the above to pie shell and return to oven.   Bake at 350 degrees for 45 miutes.

Recipe 76 ———————————————

Nut Butter Balls

In a large bowl mix the following:

3 cups maple syrup

1 cup Sucanat sugar

4 tsp. rose water or water

2 cups walnuts (chopped)

3 cups almond butter

6 cups whole-wheat pastry flour

Mix and roll into balls the size of a quarter.   Roll with coconut flour.

Place on tray lined with parchment paper or cookie mat.

Bake at 350 degrees for 25 minutes.

Recipe 77 ───────────────────────

Sharareh Shabafrooz Garlic Bread Spread - Butter

To make butter, place the following in a bowl and microwave for 5 minutes:

2/3 cup cornmeal

1/2 tsp. Bio-salt

2 cups water

Mix and set aside.

Then place all the above with the following in a Vitamix:

1 tsp. Bio-salt

½ cup water

1 cup coconut

To make garlic spread for bread, add the above to the following:

1 cup sesame seeds

1 cup cashews (cleaned)

8 tbsp. lemon juice

16 cloves garlic

2 cups water

½ tsp. Bio-salt

Mix in a bowl by hand, and add all the above with:

2 tsp. dill

2 tsp. marjoram

2 tsp. onion flakes

Spread on bread and bake at 350 degrees for 10 minutes.

Recipe 78

Glazed Carrot Cake

Frosting: Place the following in a Vitamix or blender:

1 cup maple syrup

1 cup almond butter

½ cup tofu

4 tsp. sifted whole-wheat pastry flour

1 tsp. cinnamon

½ tsp. Bio-salt

Set aside.

Cake: Toast ½ cup sunflower seeds, and then add the following to a bowl:

1 cup sifted whole-wheat pastry flour

1 cup shredded carrots

1 cup maple syrup

Mix and add 1 tbsp. yeast into ¼ cup of finger-warm water; let sit until dough rises.

Place in a pan, and bake at 350 degrees for 30 minutes.

Use the toothpick test to make sure the center is done.

Remove from oven and place glaze on top cake and then return to the oven for ten more minutes.

Recipe 79 ———————————————————

Waffles With Cashews And Oatmeal

Place in a Vitamix or blender the following:

9 cups water

6 cups oatmeal

1/3 cup cashews

1 tbsp. maple syrup or 1 tbsp. Sucanat sugar

    Cook in waffle iron for 12 to 13 minutes.

Recipe 80 _____

Lemon Pineapple Pie

Place in a Vitamix:

¼ cup plus 1 tbsp. tapioca flour

½ cup lemon juice

Mix and add:

2 cups maple syrup

¼ tsp. Bio-salt

1 brick or 1 pound tofu

1 20 ounce can pineapple (drain juice)

Mix and set aside.

For crust, see special pie crust recipe #38.

Use a glass dish lined with parchment paper (9 x 12 inches).

Depending on how thick you want the crust, you may have to make one, two, or three times the pie crust recipe. Form pie crust in dish. Pour all the Vitamix ingredients into pie shell.

Bake at 350 degrees for 45 minutes.

Recipe 81

Cornbread

Mix the following in a large bowl:

4 cups warm water

4 tbsp. maple syrup

2 tsp. Bio-salt.

2 cups cornmeal

2 cups cornmeal flour

2 cups sifted whole-wheat pastry flour

Mix and let sit until mixture is room temperature, then add 1 tbsp. yeast into ¼ cup finger-warm water and let sit for two hours or until dough rises.

Mix and place in a glass dish (9 x 12 inches) lined with parchment paper.

Bake at 375 degrees for 35 to 40 minutes.

Recipe 82 ————————————————

Matt Mooney Roast For Any Holiday

In a large pan, add and sauté the following approximately 15 minutes on low:

2 chopped onions

4 long green onions cut small

1 cup olives cut each in half

2 tbsp. lemon juice

3 cups walnuts, chopped

2 tbsp. Bragg Liquid Aminos

1 shredded carrot

3 cloves garlic, cut small

2 stalks chopped celery

½ cup cilantro, cut small

2 cups water

1 cup peas

1 tsp. sage

1 tbsp. Bio-salt

½ tsp. thyme

1 tsp. marjoram

Continue to sauté and stir.

The night before, soak 2 cups rice in 4½ cups water.

The next day, bake at 350 degrees for two hours, and add to pan with one loaf of Ezekiel bread, torn by hand, each slice torn in six parts.

Mix and press (use back of large spoon) into a glass dish 9 x 12 inches, lined with parchment paper.

Bake for one hour at 350 degrees.

Recipe 83 ————————————————

Spice Doughnuts

Place the following in a Vitamix or blender:

½ cup Sucanat sugar

1 tbsp. almond butter

½ cup tofu

½ cup soymilk

½ cup maple syrup

1 tsp. Bio-salt

1 tbsp. cinnamon

Two cups sifted whole-wheat pastry flour

Let mixture sit until room temperature.

Then add 1 tbsp. yeast mixed with ¼ cup finger-warm water, and let sit for two hours or until dough rises.

Place batter in doughnut molds, filling only halfway.

Bake at 400 degrees for 10 minutes. Let cool for one hour, then add glaze.

Recipe 84 ————————————————

Spanish Rice

Place the following in a pan:

6 tomatoes cut small

Half an onion

¼ cup corn

¼ cup peas

2 tbsp. Bragg Liquid Aminos

1 bell pepper (red or green), cut small

    Boil on low for 10 to 15 minutes, and then add:

2 tbsp. oregano

2 tbsp. parsley

2 tsp. basil

2 tsp. chili powder

2 tsp. Bio-salt

    See Recipe 5.

    Add all the above to cooked rice (cooked rice should be soaked the night before) and mix.

Recipe 85

Pineapple Cookies

See butter cookie recipe 45. Must double recipe.

Place in a Vitamix or blender:

2 cans 20 ounce crushed pineapple (drain the juice)

1 tsp. vanilla

¼ tsp. Bio-salt

3 cups Sucanat sugar

Grind 2 to 3 cups walnuts and set aside.

THE DOUGH:

Roll out the dough and use a circular cookie cutter, 2-inch circle, and place one spoonful of fruit inside the circle in the center. Then sprinkle walnuts (one tsp.) on top of mixture.   Place another circle on top to form a sandwich and pinch sides together. Poke with a fork to let air inside.

You can make the dough and fruit the night before.

Bake at 375 degrees for 20 minutes.

Recipe 86 _____

Carob Cupcakes

See butter cookie recipe 45.

Add to the dough ½ cup carob and ½ cup Roma. Cut recipe to only half. Makes approximately 3 dozen.

Roll out the dough and use a round cookie cutter, 4 inches. Place cookie circle into cupcake holder, but do not press into holder. Place in a cupcake pan. For the filling inside, see Parvin Malek recipe 40.

Place filling inside the cupcake shell. Then place in pan. You can add coconut to the top before placing it in the oven.

Bake at 375 degrees for 20 minutes.

Recipe 87

Any Fruit Cup Cookie

For dough: use butter cookie recipe 45.

Use cupcake holders and cupcake pan.   Boil fruit until thick, for 1½ hours on warm.   Then add 2 tbsp. tapioca, then boil another half hour and let cool.   See any fruit pie recipe.

Roll out the dough and use a round cookie cutter, 4 inches. Place circle into cupcake holder, but do not press into holder.   Then place in a cupcake pan.

Place fruit inside, approximately half-full, and then sprinkle one tbsp. walnuts (ground).

Bake at 375 degrees for 20 minutes.

Recipe 88 _____

Setareh Tais Cake

Using the 8 piece roman column, separate sets, 18 inch plate

See the following recipes:

Whipped cream, see recipe 170.
For cake, see recipe 72.
Carob glaze, see recipe 23.
Carob doughnuts, see recipe 52.

Use parchment paper inside cake pan.

Bake at 325 degrees for 50 minutes.

Use the toothpick test to see if center is done.

This is a product made by Walton Enterprises, which includes two plates 18 inch x 18 inch held up by roman columns pillars. See any cooking supply or store that sells cake supplies.

Recipe 89

Carob Date Pistachio Pastry

CRUST: In a large bowl, mix the following:

2 cups maple syrup

1/3 cup roasted pistachios

1/3 cup roasted pistachios (chopped or ground)

1/3 cup Roma powder

1/3 cup carob powder

2 tbsp. tapioca flour

2 cups almond butter

5 cups sifted whole-wheat pastry flour

Mix and set aside 2 cups of this mixture.

In a cookie tray lined with parchment paper, form this dough into a crust. Do not use a flat cookie tray.

TOPPING:

Mix in another bowl:

2 cups of the above mixture

2 cups maple syrup

3 cups dates cut small

1/3 cup pistachio nuts (roasted)

And another 1/3 cup pistachio nuts (roasted)

Place this topping on the unbaked crust and bake at 350 degrees for 20 minutes.

In a small bowl, mix:

2 tsp. almond butter

1 cup maple syrup

¼ cup carob

¼ cup Roma

Then place on top of topping after removing above from the oven. Let cool and place in the refrigerator.

Recipe 90

Fruitcake Cookies

Place the following in a Vitamix or blender:

1 cup soymilk

1 cup maple syrup

1 tsp. vanilla

1 tsp. Bio-salt

½ cup Sucanat sugar

1 cup almond butter

1 tsp. cinnamon

½ cup tofu

Place all the above in a bowl and then add:

2½ cups sifted whole-wheat pastry flour

4 cups pecans (ground)

4 cups walnuts (ground)

1 cup papaya (dried) cut small

8 cups dates cut small

3 cups sliced dried pineapple

On a cookie sheet lined with parchment paper, form cookies into circles and bake at 350 degrees for 20 minutes.

Recipe 91

Baked Millet

Soak overnight three cups millet in a large baking bowl with:

3 tsp. Bio-salt

12 cups water

The next day, stir and bake for 2½ hours at 350 degrees.

Recipe 92

Biscotti

Place the following in a Vitamix or blender:

1 brick tofu (or 1 pound)

3 cups maple syrup

4 tsp. vanilla

4 tsp. rose water

½ tsp. Bio-salt

4 tsp. almond butter

2 tbsp. Roma

2 tbsp. carob

Mix and pour in a large bowl. Add 9-10 cups whole-wheat pastry flour, sifted. Dough should be firm. Roll into four logs on Sucanat sugar, approximately 1 to 2 cups. Lay four logs on a cookie tray lined with parchment paper. Bake at 350 degrees for 5 to 10 minutes. Remove from oven and cut diagonally then return to oven for 12 to 15 minutes.

Recipe 93 ———————————————————

Multigrain Crackers

The night before, mix in bags all dry ingredients and clean trays.

Place the following in a Vitamix or blender:

4 cups water

4 tbsp. Bio-salt

1 tsp. onion power

1 tsp. caraway seeds.

1 cup corn flour

1 cup oatmeal flour

1 cup buckwheat flour

1 cup rye flour

1 tsp. garlic powder

4 tbsp. millet flour

1 cup barley flour

One recipe makes four trays of crackers. Batter is very thick; spread on a cookie sheet very thinly with a plastic knife.

First grind the following and then sprinkle on top of crackers:

poppy seeds

sunflower seeds

pumpkin seeds

Bake at 350 degrees for five minutes; remove from oven and with a plastic knife, cut on tray cracker-size squares. Return to oven for 20 minutes or until baked.

General Information

Do not drink any liquids while eating meals. Drink all the water you want a half hour before eating, none during eating, and all the water you want two hours after eating.

This is not a restriction. I drink one to two and a half gallons daily, and in the summer, I drink up to three gallons a day. Eat two meals daily; do not mix fruits and vegetables together. This is not a restriction, and not hard to accomplish. The purpose this information is to avoid digestive disorders and achieve radiant health.

Dessert: One-quarter pound one time a day, to be consumed directly after the meal.

All meals are consumed within one hour, and not less than half an hour. Otherwise you are not chewing long enough.

Cleaning the colon is very necessary. One hour each, total of six sessions consecutively. See a colon hydrotherapist. I recommend this to be done after you start eating healthily.

Conclusion

Eating junk food is very expensive and will cost you a loss of a good life, which you cannot afford.

I urge you to not to be involved in this path. It is so easy, fun, and rewarding to treat your body right. Start with these delicious recipes and the information contained within this book. Get your body cleaned by hydrotherapy. The changes will not be temporary, and will be very obvious within fourteen days. You will see tremendous results in a positive manner. My entire life has changed and I am free, no longer sick. What was impossible is now possible by changing. I do not have the limitations a sick body to hold me back.

It does not take a crystal ball or a college education to figure out where a person is headed, if their body continues to be mistreated. But it does take common sense.

Please do not copy or give away any material, not just because it is copyright-protected material, but doing this will interfere with my program of feeding and educating the unhealthy. Instead, my wish is that you share your cooking with friends, family, and strangers.

Questions, concerns, and suggestions are welcomed.
24-hour message phone: 559-435-4069
This line will also have some general information, updates, Web sites, and future information.

Want a recipe named after you or a friend? The cost is $2,600.
Want an autographed book? Price is to be announced on Web site.

To order or inquire about the Cellerciser™
Call 1-800-856-4863
For a substantial discount, mention my name.

References

Frederick Mikel Huck: Author, researcher, *Weight Loss Your Body Will Accept*

Dr. Ede Koenig: President and founder of The Radiant Health Institute. Author of *The Whole Kernel*

Dr. Windell Stanley Kirby: Eminent virologist, Nobel Prize 1957. *Dangers of Eating Animal Products*

Recipe List

1. BAKED POTATO

2. SALADS

3. PASTA

4. PASTA SAUCE - TOMATO SAUCE

5. BROWN RICE

6. TEXAN RICE

7. BELL PEPPER RICE

8. TOSTADAS

9. POPCORN

10. HOT SAUCE

11. CINDY HUCK BEANS FOR BURRITOS

12. TODD NEUMILLER CHINESE SOUP

13. ALMOND BUTTER

14. PIZZA SAUCE

15. PIZZA DOUGH (FOR PIES)

16. WAFFLES

17. TAMALE CASSEROLE

18. MAPLE SYRUP CAKE

19. PAN-FRIED NOODLES

20. FRUIT ICING

21. CAROB BAKED ALASKA

22. VANILLA CAKE

23. CAROB GLAZE

24. MAPLE OATMEAL CAKE

25. CLOVE COOKIES

26. DONALD W. HUCK COCONUT COOKIES

27. CAROB ROMA OATMEAL COOKIES

28. DEEP-DISH PIZZA

29. COCONUT OATMEAL CAROB ROMA COOKIES

30. COCONUT OATMEAL COOKIES

31. CAROB ROMA COCONUT OATMEAL WHOLE-WHEAT PASTRY FLOUR COOKIES

32. COCONUT OATMEAL WHOLE-WHEAT PASTRY FLOUR COOKIES

33. STUFFED BELL PEPPERS

34. MAPLE SYRUP COOKIES

35. CAROB COOKIES

36. CAROB BROWN CAKE

37. ANY FRUIT COOKIES (PEACH, CHERRY, APRICOT)

38. SPECIAL PIE CRUST

39. PUMPKIN PIE

40. PARVIN MALEK CAROB PIE

41. ALMOND BUTTER COOKIES 2

42. CAROB FILLING

43. EVELYN ANN MENZIE OLD-FASHIONED GLAZE

44. PINEAPPLE PIE

45. BUTTER COOKIES

46. SUCANAT COOKIES

47. INEZ A. MENZIE COCONUT COOKIES

48. TURNOVERS

49. GOLDEN MACAROONS

50. ORIENTAL CRUNCH

51. PINEAPPLE CANDY

52. CAROB DOUGHNUTS

53. LEMON DOUGHNUTS

54. GRAIN PIZZA

55. CORNMEAL PIZZA

56. CAROB BROWNIES

57. ROBERT E. MENZIE WALNUT PIE

58. APRICOT COCONUT WALNUT SQUARES

59. PISTACHIO SCONES

60. EGG ROLLS

61. ROASTED SALTED NUTS

62. FUDGE CUP COOKIE

63. FUDGE SAUCE

64. PINEAPPLE COOKIES

65. TAMALE BEAN PIE

66. NUT PIE

67. DATE WALNUT COOKIES

68. CARAMELIZED GINGER HAZELNUT TART

69. PAPAYA COOKIES

70. CAJUN MIXED NUTS

71. TACO SALAD SHELLS

72. FOR CAKE - WEDDING-STYLE CAKE

73. SPANISH MILLET CASSEROLE

74. ENCHILADAS

75. CAROB PIE

76. NUT BUTTER BALLS

77. SHARAREH SHABAFROOZ GARLIC BREAD SPREAD/BUTTER

78. GLAZED CARROT CAKE

79. WAFFLES WITH CASHEWS AND OATMEAL

80. LEMON PINEAPPLE PIE

81. CORNBREAD

82. MATTHEW F. MOONEY ROAST FOR ANY HOLIDAY

83. SPICE DOUGHNUTS

84. SPANISH RICE

85. PINEAPPLE SANDWICH COOKIE

86. CAROB CUP COOKIE

87. ANY FRUIT CUP COOKIE

88. SETAREH TAIS CAKE

89. CAROB DATE PISTACHIO PASTRY

90. FRUITCAKE COOKIE

91. BAKED MILLET

92. BISCOTTI

93. MULTIGRAIN CRACKERS

94. POT PIE

95. BASIC COOKIE WITH FROSTING

96. TACO SHELLS

97. ANY FRUIT PASTRY

98. PINEAPPLE FROSTING

99. PINEAPPLE UPSIDE-DOWN CAKE

100. HOT BEANS FOR BURRITOS

101. APRICOT PIE

102. APPLE PIE

103. PLUM PIE

104. PIZZA SAUCE NO. 3

105. PIZZA SAUCE NO. 1

106. COFFEE MUFFINS

107. GLORIA DUGGINS PECAN CANDY

108. PETER P. PANAGOPOULOS ALMOND FUDGE

109. PETE/ROSA CERRILLO CINNAMON WALNUT CANDY

110. SUGARED NUTS

111. PAPAYA CANDY

112. CAROB CAKE

113. THELMA MAIN HAZELNUT FUDGE

114. WHEAT CORNMEAL PIZZA

115. MARGARET/HARVEY BINDER PECAN FUDGE

116. MICHAEL F. MOONEY PECAN ROMA CAROB CANDY

117. BELLE HUCK WALNUT FUDGE

118. SAUCE FOR INSIDE CINNAMON ROLLS

119. NECTARINE PIE

120. COOKIES/CAROB PLAIN OR ROMA

121. CAROB BARS

122. SPICE BUTTER COOKIES

123. OAT CRACKERS

124. CINNAMON SUGAR DOUGHNUT TOPPING

125. JELLY DOUGHNUT FILLING

126. STRUDEL DOUGH

127. DATE CUP COOKIE

128. ITALIAN SAUCE

129 LASAGNA

130. BOB PANAGOPOULOS PIZZA SAUCE NO. 2

131. CUBAN BLACK BEANS IN RICE

132. BLACK BEANS

133. LIGHT FUDGE

134. DARK FUDGE

135. PIGEON BEANS

136. XENIA PANAGOPOULOS PIGEON RICE

137. ALEXANDRA PANAGOPOULOS SWEET AND SOUR SAUCE NO. 1

138. INEZ SPEIDELL SWEET AND SOUR SAUCE NO. 2

139. VERY VERY HOT SAUCE

140. LENTILS

141. SHRIMP SAUCE

142. GABRIEL CERRILLO ALMOND CAROB CANDY

143. CAROB ROMA CANDY

144. WALNUT CINNAMON CLUSTERS

145. TAMARA NEUMILLER SPANISH PASTA

146. CHINESE RICE

147. CHILI BEANS

148. TAMALES

149. VEGETABLE SOUP

150. CAROB ROMA COOKIES

151. RAY AND LINDA PANAGOPOULOS SUNFLOWER COCONUT WAFFLES

152. WAFFLES, OATMEAL, AND ALMONDS

153. RHI CAROB AND ROMA OATMEAL WWP NUTLESS COOKIE

154. HOT SAUCE

155. RED BEANS FOR TOP OF RICE

156. CORNMEAL WAFFLES

186. CAROB COCONUT FROSTING

187. SPECIAL SEASONING FOR ANYTHING

188. ITALIAN SALAD DRESSING

189. PINEAPPLE ICE CREAM

190. ORANGE ICE CREAM

191. CATSUP EXTRA

192. CHERRY ICE CREAM

193. THESE COLORS TO BE USED WITH WHIPPED CREAM (SEE RECIPE NO. 170) REAL COLORS FOR CAKES AND COOKIES

194. CAROB PUDDING OR PIE FILLING

195. ENGLISH TOFFEE COOKIE

196. CAROB CAKE FROSTING

197. COCONUT CAKE

198. PUMPKIN COOKIES

199. MARSELLAS PANAGOPOULOS BRAZIL NUT ICE CREAM

200. TAHEREH MALEK PUMPKIN ICE CREAM

201. BAKED BROWN RICE

202. GINGER CANDY

203. SANDY MOONEY COFFEE CAKE

204. PAPAYA WALNUT COOKIES

205. LEMON CARROT COOKIES

206. CAROB SANDWICH COOKIES

207. DAISY FROSTING

208. BLACK-EYED PEAS

209. ALMOND BUTTER FROSTING

210. CRUNCH TOPPING FOR ANY BAKED PIE

211. CHERI GILBERT COOKED CAROB GLAZE

212. SUCANAT SUGAR GLAZE

213. ROMA CREAM FROSTING

214. LEMON FILLING

215. BAR-B-QUE SAUCE

216. TOFU FROSTING

217. SWEET SUGAR ICING

218. BLACK-EYED PEAS IN RICE

219. SOYMILK CORNBREAD

220. OATMEAL ALMOND COOKIE

221. SPICED CUPCAKES

222. DATE OATMEAL COOKIE

223. ORANGE COCONUT COOKIE

224. DATE COOKIE BAR

225. APRICOT COOKIE BAR

226. GINGER PANCAKES

227. LEMON PASTRY

228. LEMON SUGAR COOKIES

229. DATE BROWNIES

230. ORIGINAL SALT WATER TAFFY

231. AURA VICTORIA HUCK PEPPERMINT SALT WATER TAFFY

232. LEMON SALT WATER TAFFY

233. VANILLA SALT WATER TAFFY

234. ORANGE SALT WATER TAFFY

235. JACK PANAGOPOULOS ROMA SALT WATER TAFFY

236. ADRIANA CERRILLO PECAN SALT WATER TAFFY

237. ELMER LYLE MENZIE ALMOND SALT WATER TAFFY

238. ASHLEY SPEIDELL WALNUT SALT WATER TAFFY

239. ROSS H. MENZIE CAROB SALT WATER TAFFY

240. COCONUT SALT WATER TAFFY

241. CINNAMON SALT WATER TAFFY

242. GINGER SALT WATER TAFFY

243. GENE KOENIG ENGLISH TOFFEE CANDY

244. LUCILLE GILBERT LEMON CHEESECAKE

245. ORANGE CHEESECAKE

246. ASHER MICHAEL NEUMILLER CAROB CHEESECAKE

247. ALLIE NICOLE BLUMA NEUMILLER CAROB CAKE

248. DR. EDE VANILLA SUGAR CAKE

249. WALNUT SQUARE COOKIES

250. TARA SHABAFROOZ PECAN SQUARE COOKIES

251. ALMOND SQUARE COOKIES

252. MARGRET ANN MENZIE PECAN ROPE COOKIES

253. MASSOOD SHABAFROOZ WALNUT ROPE COOKIES

254. ALMOND ROPE COOKIES

255. RHI COCONUT OATMEAL CAROB AND ROMA COOKIES

256. RHI COCONUT OATMEAL COOKIES

257. RHI COCONUT OATMEAL WHOLE-WHEAT PASTRY FLOUR COOKIES

258. RHI CAROB COCONUT COOKIES

259. RHI COCONUT COOKIES

260. RHI CAROB AND ROMA OATMEAL COOKIES

261. RHI VANILLA DOUGHNUTS OR CAKE

262. RHI CAROB BROWN CAKE

263. RHI GOLDEN MACAROONS

264. RHI COFFEE MUFFINS

265. RHI SPICED CUPCAKES

266. PEPPERMINT WALNUT FUDGE

267. PEPPERMINT ICE CREAM

268. CAROB AND ROMA ICE CREAM

269. CHERRY FUDGE

270. CAROB ROMA PEPPERMINT ICE CREAM

271. PEACH APRICOT PIE

272. ROMA BAKED ALASKA

273. RAISIN BAR COOKIES

274. FREDERICK HUCK POCKET BREAD FOLDING DIAGRAM

275. NOOSHIN MALEK SEE MOUSEH

276. ZOHREH EHSANI BLUEBERRY ICE CREAM

277. POCKET PIZZA ONE

278. RAISIN CREAM PIE

279. DR. EDE KOENIG BEEROCK

280. DATE CREAM PIE

281. POCKET RAISIN PASTRY

282. POCKET PIZZA 3

283. POCKET PIZZA 4

284. POCKET PIZZA 2

285. POCKET DATE PASTRY

286. POCKET PLUM PASTRY

287. PLUM CREAM PIE

288. POCKET CAROB PASTRY

289. POCKET ROMA PASTRY

290. POCKET WALNUT PASTRY

291. POCKET APRICOT PASTRY

292. POCKET CHERRY PASTRY

293. POCKET PEACH PASTRY

294. POCKET PINEAPPLE-LEMON PASTRY

295. POCKET PUMPKIN PASTRY

296. POCKET APPLE PASTRY

297. POCKET EGG ROLLS

298. POCKET BEAN BURRITO

299. APRICOT CREAM PIE

300. VERA WAIVSCHIDT CHERRY CREAM PIE

301. PEACH CREAM PIE

302. APPLE CREAM PIE

303. TAHEREH TAHERIAN HABANERO HOT SAUCE

304. SHAHNAZ SHAINEE HOT AND SPICY PINTO BEANS

305. PAYAM MALEK ZADEH CAROB WHEAT COOKIES

306. RAISIN ICE CREAM

307. TOMATO CASSEROLE

308. RAISIN FACE COOKIE

309. DATE FACE COOKIE

310. PINEAPPLE COCONUT SQUARES

311. ORANGE PINEAPPLE ICE CREAM

312. LEMON PINEAPPLE ICE CREAM

313. ROMA FACE COOKIE

314. CAROB FACE COOKIE

315. PUMPKIN FACE COOKIE

316. PINEAPPLE FACE COOKIE

317. APPLE FACE COOKIE

318. PEACH FACE COOKIE

319. APRICOT FACE COOKIE

320. PLUM FACE COOKIE

321. CHERRY FACE COOKIE

322. WALNUT DOME COOKIES

323. ALMOND DOME COOKIES

324. PECAN DOME COOKIES

325. CAROB DOME COOKIES

326. ROMA DOME COOKIES

327. COFFEE CUP COOKIE

328. RAISIN CUP COOKIE

329. WALNUT CUP COOKIE

330. POCKET PASTA NO. 4

331. POCKET PASTA NO. 2

332. POCKET PASTA NO. 3

333. POCKET PASTA NO. 1

334. BRAZIL NUT CARAMEL CANDY

335. HABANERO BAKED RICE

336. MACADAMIA CARAMEL CANDY

337. CINNAMON CARAMEL CANDY

338. WALNUT CARAMEL CANDY

339. COCONUT CARAMEL CANDY

340. PECAN CARAMEL CANDY

341. PISTACHIO CARAMEL CANDY

342. HAZEL NUT CARAMEL CANDY

343. CASHEW CARAMEL CANDY

344. ROASTED ALMOND CARAMEL CANDY

345. LEMON CARAMEL CANDY

346. ORANGE CARAMEL CANDY

347. CAROB CARAMEL CANDY

348. ROMA CARAMEL CANDY

349. PEPPERMINT CARAMEL CANDY

350. GINGER CARAMEL CANDY

351. HERBS & GARLIC BAKED RICE

352. WALNUT & ALMOND FROSTING

353. PINEAPPLE & LEMON GLAZE

354. ROMA TOFU COOKIES

355. CAROB TOFU COOKIES

356. CINNAMON TOFU COOKIES

357. RAISIN TOFU COOKIES

358. APRICOT TOFU COOKIES

359. DATE TOFU COOKIES

360. CRANBERRY TOFU COOKIES

361. SPICE TOFU COOKIES

362. PAPAYA TOFU COOKIES

363. COCONUT TOFU COOKIES

364. LEMON TOFU COOKIES

365. ORANGE TOFU COOKIES

366. PINEAPPLE TOFU COOKIES

367. BLACK BEAN SOUP

368. LEMON COCONUT COOKIES

369. CHERRY SUGAR COOKIES

370. ORANGE SUGAR COOKIES

371. RAISIN SUGAR COOKIES

372. ROMA SUGAR COOKIES

373. APPLE SUGAR COOKIES

374. CAROB SUGAR COOKIES

375. PEPPERMINT SUGAR COOKIES

376. BLUEBERRY SUGAR COOKIES

377. DATE SUGAR COOKIES

378. PINEAPPLE SUGAR COOKIES

379. PLUM SUGAR COOKIES

380. PEACH SUGAR COOKIES

381. APRICOT SUGAR COOKIES

382. NECTARINE SUGAR COOKIES

383. CRANBERRY SUGAR COOKIES

384. PUMPKIN SUGAR COOKIES

385. COCONUT CAROB CARAMEL CANDY

386. COCONUT LEMON CARAMEL CANDY

387. COCONUT CINNAMON CARAMEL CANDY
388. COCONUT ORANGE CARAMEL CANDY
389. COCONUT PEPPERMINT CARAMEL CANDY
390. COCONUT ROMA CARAMEL CANDY
391. COCONUT GINGER CARAMEL CANDY
392. DATE OATMEAL COOKIES
393. RAISIN OATMEAL COOKIES
394. WALNUT DATE COOKIES
395. WALNUT LEMON COOKIES
396. WALNUT RAISIN COOKIES
397. WALNUT ORANGE COOKIES
398. WALNUT CHERRY COOKIES
399. COCONUT DATE COOKIES
400. COCONUT CHERRY COOKIES
401. COCONUT RAISIN COOKIES
402. ONION DRIED ROASTED NUTS
403. GARLIC DRIED ROASTED NUTS
404. HABANERO DRIED ROASTED NUTS
405. CAYENNE DRIED ROASTED NUTS
406. BLACK BEAN RICE
407. SALTED-HABANERO DRIED ROASTED NUT MIX
408. MAPLE SYRUP DRIED ROASTED NUTS
409. CAROB MACAROONS
410. LEMON MACAROONS
411. ROMA MACAROONS
412. ORANGE MACAROONS
413. PEPPERMINT FROSTING
414. PINEAPPLE-LEMON BAKED ALASKA
415. LEMON BAKED ALASKA

416. ORANGE BAKED ALASKA

417. PEPPERMINT BAKED ALASKA

418. VANILLA BAKED ALASKA

419. RED HOT FIRE SAUCE

420. APRICOT ICE CREAM

421. TWICE-COOKED HERB POTATO

422. PEPPERMINT MACAROONS

423. PEACH ICE CREAM

424. TWICE-COOKED SPICY POTATO

425. PLUM MACAROONS

426. SPICY GARLIC SPREAD

427. ITALIAN SPREAD

428. WALNUT WAFFLES

429. POPPY SEED WAFFLES

430. PUMPKIN SEED WAFFLES

431. CAROB SUCANAT SUGAR COOKIES

432. ROMA SUCANAT SUGAR COOKIES

433. PEPPERMINT SUCANAT SUGAR COOKIES

434. CINNAMON SUCANAT SUGAR COOKIES

435. GINGER SUCANAT SUGAR COOKIES

436. CAROB SUGARED NUTS

437. ROMA SUGARED NUTS

438. PECAN PIE

439. BLUEBERRY CREAM PIE

440. GRAPE PIE